Slim Down, Shape Up

A Short Guide To Sustainable Weight Loss

By

Alisha Patterson

Copyright © Alisha Patterson 2023. All rights reserved

Table Of Contents

Slim Down, Shape Up

Introduction:

It can be difficult to keep a healthy weight in today's society where fast food and sedentary activities are the norms. We all understand, though, that being overweight increases our risk for a number of health issues, such as diabetes, heart disease, and even some types of cancer, in addition to how we look physically.

There are innumerable books, programs, and supplements that promise simple and quick results in the enormous diet and weight loss business. Yet in reality, a lot of these materials and strategies are unsustainable and might even be hazardous to your health. Here's where Slim Down, Shape Up comes in. This book is created to give you all the tools and knowledge you need to achieve your weight loss goals and maintain a healthy lifestyle, without turning to fad diets or unhealthy habits.

This book does not provide a quick fix or a crash diet. Instead, it provides a thorough manual for long-term weight loss that focuses on implementing simple, healthy lifestyle adjustments. The goal is to assist you in achieving and maintaining a healthy weight for life.

Many facets of weight loss are covered in Slim Down, Shape Up, including diet, exercise, attitude, and habit creation. You will discover how to prepare nutritious meals and snacks, select the best workouts for your body type and level of fitness, and cultivate a positive outlook that will keep you motivated and on track.

Slim Down, Shape Up will be your go-to resource for reaching your weight reduction objectives, whether you're hoping to shed a few pounds or start a complete transformation. You may finally bid dangerous weight reduction methods and crash diets farewell with this book as your guide, and say hello to a healthier, happier you!

Chapter 1

The Science Of Losing Weight: Knowing What Your Body Needs

The subject of weight loss is complicated and involves several variables, including the consumption of macronutrients and metabolism. We'll delve into the science of weight loss in this chapter, learning about the fundamentals of metabolism and the various elements that can influence your body's capacity to burn fat.

The concept of calories is among the most crucial to comprehend when it comes to weight loss. Your body needs a specific number of calories per day to function correctly, so calories can be thought of as a unit of energy. You will put on weight if you eat more calories than your body requires. You will lose weight if you consume fewer calories than your body requires.

Naturally, it's not quite that easy. Your body's capacity to burn fat can be impacted by a number of variables, including your metabolism, hormone levels, and degree of activity. For instance, in order to lose the same amount of weight, a person with a slower metabolism might need to consume fewer calories than a person with a faster metabolism.

To create a personalized weight loss plan that is effective for you, you must first understand the needs of your body. You can make sure that you are giving your body the proper balance of nutrients to meet your goals by estimating your daily calorie needs and monitoring your macronutrient consumption.

Chapter 2

Developing A Good Attitude For Long-Lasting Results

In order to lose weight, having the right mindset is crucial. We'll examine how goal-setting, self-talk, and visualization can all support your weight loss efforts.

Negative self-talk is one of the main obstacles to successful weight loss. A lot of us struggle with an inner voice that tells us we're not good enough or that we'll never succeed in our endeavors. This kind of thinking can be quite harmful since it can make us feel self-conscious and undermine our efforts to lose weight.

It's crucial to engage in positive self-talk in order to combat negative self-talk. This entails changing your negative ideas to positive ones and putting more emphasis on your strengths than your faults. Visualization is a potent technique for weight loss since it may inspire and motivate you as you picture yourself succeeding in your endeavors.

Setting goals is yet another crucial component of having a positive outlook. Throughout your weight loss journey, you can boost your confidence and stay motivated by setting clear, attainable goals and monitoring your progress.

Chapter 3

Making A Healthy Eating Plan: Nutrition For Weight Loss

A crucial element of weight loss is nutrition. We'll concentrate on the fundamentals of healthy eating, including the value of whole foods, portion control, and hydration.

Not all calories are created equal, which is among the most crucial considerations when it comes to diet for weight loss. While eating fewer calories than your body requires to lose weight is crucial, you should also concentrate on eating nutrient-dense foods that will keep you feeling content and full.

A healthy diet is built on entire foods including fruits, vegetables, lean proteins, and whole grains. These meals are typically lower in calories than processed foods and offer a variety of critical nutrients, including fiber, vitamins, and minerals.

Controlling portions is essential for successful weight loss. You may prevent overeating and taking more calories than your body requires by calculating your meals and engaging in mindful eating.

And finally, staying hydrated is crucial for losing weight. Staying hydrated and reducing cravings are just a few benefits of drinking lots of water. It also makes you feel full and satisfied.

Chapter 4

How To Create A Balanced Plate With Protein

Protein is a necessary food that is important for weight loss. The advantages of protein, how to estimate your protein requirements, and how to include protein in your meals are all covered in this chapter.

One of the main advantages of protein is that it makes you feel happy and full, which can lower cravings and lead to a reduction in overall calorie intake. Protein is also necessary for maintaining a healthy metabolism and achieving a leaner body composition since it helps to grow and repair muscular tissue.

Your body weight, amount of activity, and goals all be taken into consideration when determining your protein requirements. 0.8

grams of protein per pound of body weight per day is the basic norm for most people. But, this sum may change based on your particular requirements.

Focus on lean sources of protein, such as chicken, turkey, fish, beans, and lentils, to add more protein to your meals. These foods are a perfect supplement to any weight loss strategy because they are low in calories and high in protein. If you're having trouble getting enough protein from whole meals, you can also add supplements like protein powders or bars.

Chapter 5

Exercise For Weight Loss: Finding An Activity You Enjoy

A crucial element of weight loss is exercise. We'll discuss the advantages of exercise, how to make an exercise schedule, and how to locate a hobby in this chapter.

The ability to burn more calories and create a calorie deficit more quickly is one of exercise's key advantages. Exercise is also necessary for preserving a healthy metabolism, gaining lean muscle mass, and enhancing general health. Start by choosing enjoyable activities and setting reasonable goals before creating an exercise plan. This could entail cardio, weightlifting, yoga, or a mix of various exercises. Also, it's critical to mix up your workouts to avoid getting bored and make sure your body is being put to a variety of challenges.

Start out cautiously and build up the length and intensity of your workouts if you're new to exercising. To make sure you're employing proper form and technique, you might also think about working with a personal trainer or enrolling in a fitness class.

Chapter 6

The Impact Of Stress And Sleep On Your Weight Loss Journey

Stress and sleep are two elements that can significantly affect weight reduction. The relationship between sleep, stress, and weight reduction will be discussed in this chapter, along with suggestions for making improvements in each area.

Weight gain is one of the many detrimental health implications of sleep deprivation. Lack of sleep causes your body to create more ghrelin, a hormone that increases appetite, and less leptin, a hormone that makes you feel full and content. Lack of sleep can also lead to higher levels of the stress hormone cortisol, which can encourage fat storage and hinder weight loss.

Try to build a regular sleep schedule and a tranquil sleeping environment in your bedroom to enhance your sleep patterns. This can entail using blackout curtains, switching off gadgets before bed, and maintaining a cool, dark bedroom.

Another element that may affect weight reduction is stress. Your body creates more cortisol when you're under stress, which can increase appetite and cause overeating. Stress can also trigger emotional eating, which can undermine weight loss efforts.

Try incorporating stress-relieving practices into your daily schedules, such as yoga, deep breathing, or meditation. To address any underlying issues that might be generating stress, you might also think about meeting with a therapist or counselor.

Chapter 7

Progress Monitoring: Why It Matters And How To Do It

A vital part of losing weight is keeping track of your progress. This chapter will cover why tracking is necessary, what to track, and successful tracking methods.

Tracking your progress is important for many reasons, including accountability and motivation. It can be tremendously inspiring and supportive to observe success over time as you work toward your weight loss target. Also, tracking enables you to spot areas where your diet or exercise routine may need to be modified.

There are numerous alternatives accessible when it comes to tracking. You might decide to keep tabs on your dietary consumption, physical activity, body measurements, or weight. It's crucial to pick a strategy you can continue with over time and that works for you.

You can use a food journal or an app to keep track of the food you eat each day in order to monitor your calorie consumption. You can use this to spot patterns in your eating behavior and make any necessary improvements. You can keep a journal of your workouts or use a fitness tracker to monitor your exercise.

It's crucial to bear in mind that weight swings are common and can be caused by a variety of things, including water retention, muscle gain, and hormonal changes, when tracking your weight loss efforts. Consider keeping track of other indicators of improvement, such as body measurements or how your clothes fit, rather than concentrating entirely on the number on the scale.

Chapter 8:

Recovering From Setbacks And Maintaining Motivation

It can be very upsetting to hit a weight reduction plateau, which happens frequently. We'll look at why plateaus occur, how to get beyond them, and how to maintain motivation throughout your weight reduction process.

When your weight loss progress pauses in spite of your greatest efforts, a plateau occurs. Several factors, including changes in your exercise level, metabolic adjustments, or simply reaching a plateau in your calorie deficit, can cause this.

It's crucial to reevaluate your food and workout routine and make any necessary improvements in order to break through a plateau. This can entail raising your amount of activity, altering your caloric intake, or experimenting with different forms of exercise.

Maintaining motivation when trying to lose weight might be difficult. Setting achievable goals, praising yourself for accomplishments, and surrounding yourself with encouraging friends and family members can all help you stay motivated.

Chapter 9

Sustaining Weight Loss: Long-Term Success Techniques

Maintaining weight loss can be even more challenging than losing weight in the first place. We'll discuss methods for long-term weight loss success in this chapter, such as modifying one's lifestyle and setting up a support network.

Making long-term, sustainable changes to your lifestyle is one of the most effective ways to keep the weight off. This could entail focusing on full, nutrient-dense meals, finding nutritious recipes you like, and adding regular activity to your daily routine.

Building a support network might also be beneficial for keeping off weight. This could entail signing up for a support group, working out with a personal trainer, or asking friends and family for help.

In conclusion, losing weight may be a rewarding and tough experience. Making sustainable lifestyle changes calls for commitment, dedication, and a willingness to do so. In this book, we've covered a range of methods and advice for successfully losing weight, such as making a healthy food plan, working on an exercise in your daily routine, controlling stress, and getting enough sleep.

The significance of mindset and self-care in achieving weight loss success has also been covered. You may position yourself for success and maintain motivation throughout your weight loss journey by developing a positive mentality and caring for your mental and emotional well-being.

We have underlined the significance of adopting sustainable lifestyle modifications throughout this book. Although intense exercise regimens and crash diets can cause quick weight loss in the short run, they are frequently unsustainable in the long run. Instead, we advise that you put your attention toward developing a long-term, healthy lifestyle.

It's crucial to keep in mind that losing weight is a personalized process. One person's solution might not be suitable for another. It's crucial to try out several tactics to determine which suits you and your particular requirements and preferences the finest.
We've also stressed how crucial it is to look for support and direction while trying to lose weight.

Success in weight loss is attainable with the correct attitude, techniques, and encouragement. We hope that this book has given you the knowledge and motivation you need to start your own weight loss journey and reach your objectives. Always remember to applaud your progress along the road, and to be patient and nice to yourself. Wishing you luck as you work to lose weight!